Obstacle Run Training Guide

A 10 Week Program

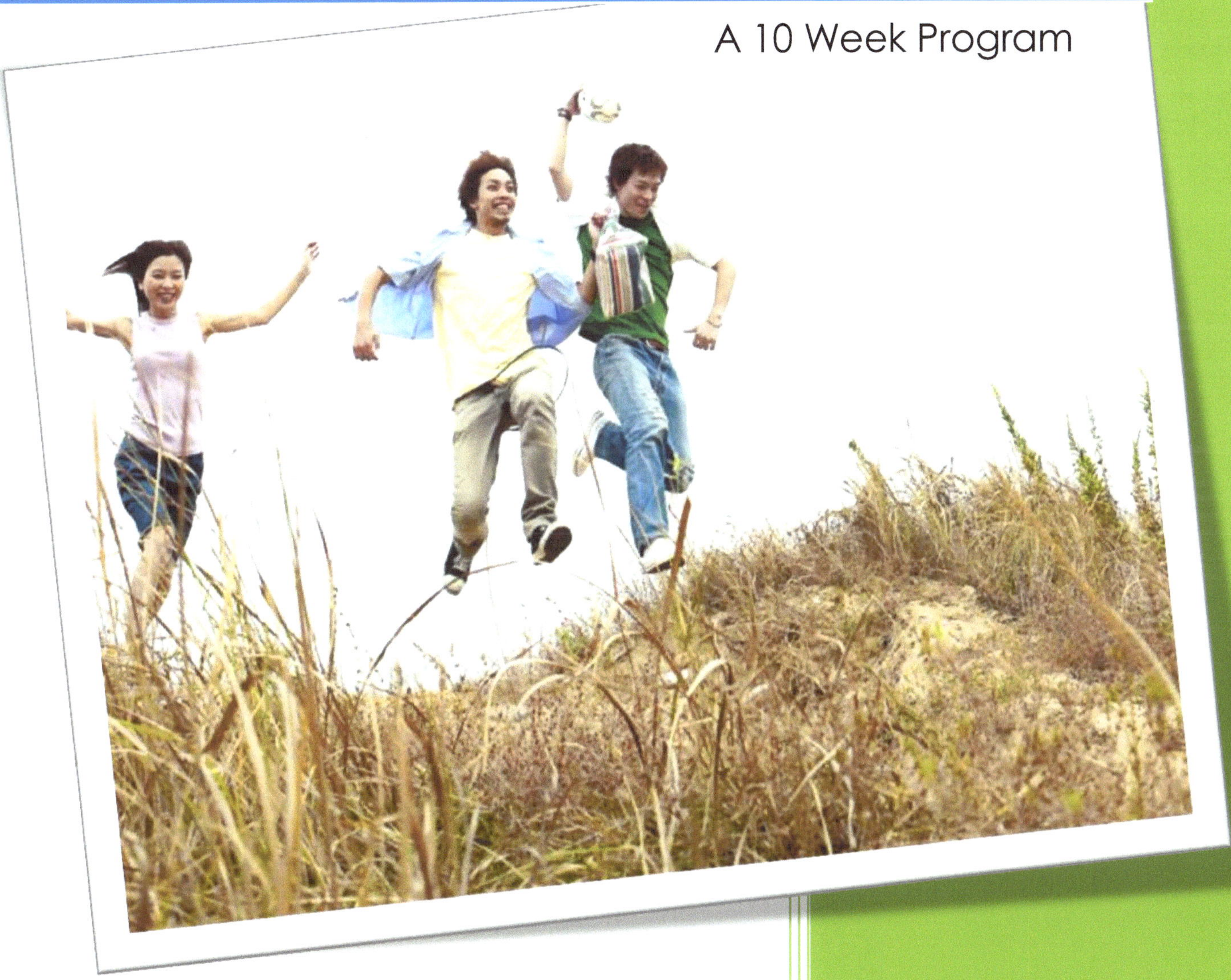

Dr. J.L. Heard

BSc, RNP, PHS, YT, PTS

Introduction

Optimal health is available for anyone who chooses to follow a natural lifestyle that incorporates exercise, whole foods and stress management. The consumption of nutrients, the air you breathe and the intellectual interactions you have all contribute in both a positive and negative way to your health. Training for any type of physical activity demands quality of these three elements to ensure your fitness at the time of the event and to prevent injury. The following Training Guide is intended to help you achieve your fitness goals in a natural, healthy way.

As with any exercise program, consult your doctor before starting. If you have any conditions or health concerns that restrict your diet, or your physical ability do not begin this plan without the approval of a medical professional. Please remember that this is a general guide and will have differing results between people. Always work at your own pace, slowing down or modifying exercises as needed.

Obstacle runs require strength, stamina and flexibility to be completed without injury. Often times multiple terrains will be crossed, there is a very different impact on the body when running over grass, sand, asphalt, cement, water, mud etc. The exercises provided will help you to increase your strength, flexibility and stamina to cross all types of terrain.

Diet

At the end of this guide you will find a few basic, healthy recipes and a chart that can be printed and filled out to track the number of servings you are consuming each day.

The ideal diet consists of 5 to 6 mini meals a day, spaced 3 to 4 hours apart, instead of 3 large meals.

A sample schedule would look like this:

7 AM	1 slice whole wheat or whole grain toast, 1 peach, ¼ cup of cottage cheese
10 AM	Celery, carrots, red & green peppers – raw, sliced & dipped in 2-3 tablespoons of unprocessed nut butter
1 PM	Salad of quinoa, sunflower seeds, and dried fruit, green leafy vegetables, drizzled with balsamic vinegar
4 PM	Whole grain crackers, fresh cheese (e.g. goat cheese), roasted red peppers
7PM	Skinless chicken breast, ½ cup steamed green beans, ½ cup steamed or raw carrots

Please note that the above sample is a guideline only, a larger man would consume more than a small woman! Also note that times are to show the spacing of meals; only eat when hungry! One of the major contributors to overeating is following pre-set times. You are unique; your body needs food at different times than someone else, depending on your physical and mental habits. Get to know your body. What are your hungry times? Some people are hungrier in the morning and can go all afternoon without food. Find your natural rhythm and go with it.

Important note: DO NOT EAT CONSTANTLY, your body needs a rest. People that munch all day are more prone to ailments. Eat a meal then wait about 3 hours before eating again. The body uses a large amount of energy to digest; depending on the foods consumed the digestion process can take 1 to 2 hours. The break allows the body to divert energy towards healing, or building up muscle.

The last meal of the day should be consumed no later than 2 hours before bed; the longer the better! During sleep the body processes slow down, remaining energy goes towards healing, both physical and mental. Your body cannot perform this much needed healing activity if it has to digest a large meal all night!

Water should be consumed throughout the day, not at meal times. Liquids consumed with meals dilute stomach acids resulting in either an overproduction of stomach acid or the under-digestion of foods. This is the main cause of an acidic stomach and/or constipation/diarrhea problems. If the body is properly hydrated throughout the day liquids will not be needed during meals, as the body will be able to produce enough saliva to facilitate swallowing. If you must have liquid with your meals slowly sip small amounts of water.

Caffeine dehydrates the body, however small amounts are okay and can even have positive health benefits. Drink no more than 1 cup of coffee or 2 cups of tea in a day. Pop and sweetened juices rob the body of nutrients, increase your caloric intake and spike blood sugar levels. These drinks should be avoided during any kind of activity, training, and for optimal health should be avoided at all times.

Carbohydrates are considered one of the most important components of a healthy diet. Complex carbohydrates are the body's main source of energy; glucose and glycogen (stored form of glucose) provide more than half of all the energy of the brain, muscles and other body tissues at any one time. When consuming please ensure good quality, whole grains, vegetables and legumes. Whole grains instead of white flours, natural sugars instead of processed or artificial.

Proteins are important for muscle production, the better quality protein you consume the faster your muscles will build. Lean proteins are recommended, stay away from fatty meats such as (processed meats, sausage, luncheon meats, pork, hamburger etc.) and consume lean meats such as chicken or turkey breast, lean cuts of beef and fresh fish. Wherever possible free range, organic animals should be consumed. Nuts and legumes are another great source of protein, though they do have a higher fat content, they are healthy fats and necessary for bodily function and brain development.

Lastly the best source of vitamins and minerals is fresh fruits and vegetables. During winter months when fresh is harder to find frozen work well too. Stay away from canned foods as the canning process breaks down nutrients. A variety of vitamins and minerals are needed for the body to build and maintain muscle, bone density and to support the nervous system. A deficiency in key nutrients can lead to muscle spasms, cramps and fatigue. Be sure to get the full range of vitamins and minerals by eating a full spectrum of colours every day. During the winter months it is beneficial to watch the discounted fruits and vegetable shelf in your supermarket. These over ripe or bruised produce are great for juicing providing a days' worth of nutrients in one tall glass.

Exercise

All exercises will be given at the beginner level with notes for any changes to be made for an intermediate level athlete. Options for workouts at home and at the gym will be provided. This guide is intended to be followed over the 10 weeks prior to an event. At the end of the guide you will find journal pages where you can record your progress.

Every week will consist of a running schedule along with strength and flexibility training. One thing most people don't realize is how important flexibility is to maneuvering an obstacle course. The best form of exercise for increasing joint and muscular flexibility is yoga. Yoga not only increases flexibility but also increases small muscle mass that supports the joints. People, men especially, are often concerned with increasing the girth of their large muscle groups. This causes strain on the joints and often leads to weakness of the small muscles resulting in injury and decreased flexibility.

Basic exercises that you will perform over the next 6weeks are: lunges, pull-ups, squats, burpees, stair climbing, running.

This guide is progressive with each week adding weight, distance and stamina. Following is a rundown of the basic form for each exercise. Further detail will be added where applicable throughout the weeks. At the 6 week mark exercises that focus more on strength will be added.

Lunges

Lunges are very important for hill climbing; they are used to strengthen the quadriceps, gluteal and hamstring muscle groups. A long lunge emphasizes the glutes whereas a short lunge emphasizes the quadriceps.

To do:

Walking lunges: Lunge forward with your left thigh parallel to the floor, bring the right leg up to meet, then lunge forward with right thigh parallel to the floor.

Switch Jump Lunges: Lunge forward with your left thigh parallel to the floor, jump up and switch leg positions, landing in a lunge with your right foot forward.

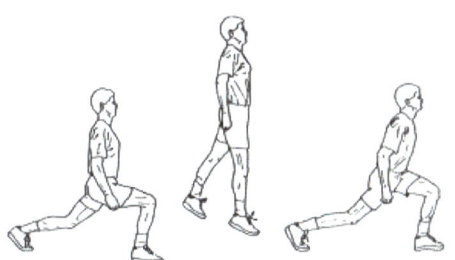
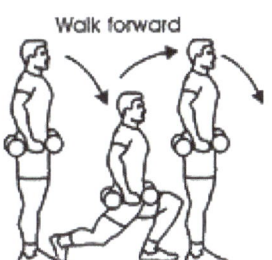

Stair Climbing

Stairs are great for cardio and leg strength. For more advanced trainers you should be running the stairs or setting a stair climber at a higher intensity.

Pull Ups

Pull ups work arms, abdominals, shoulders and chest muscle groups. Many obstacle runs have rope climbs, rings and monkey bars; pull ups will prepare you for these. If you belong to a gym many of them have *assisted pull up* machines. These are a great way for beginners to add this exercise to their workout as they balance out your body weight so that you do not have to pull your entire weight, over time you work up to unassisted pull ups. For home workouts a trx strap comes in handy for assisted pull ups.

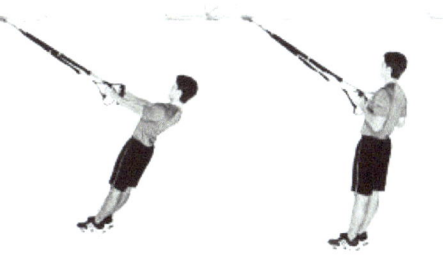

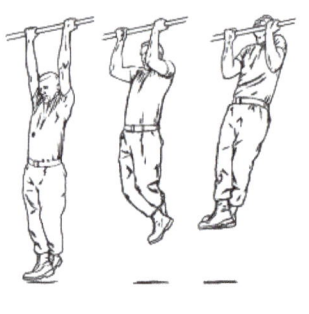

To Do:

Grip the bar with hands shoulder width apart in one of three ways; overhand, underhand, alternative-hand grip. Pull the body up until the chin clears the bar, and finish by lowering the body until your arms and shoulders are fully extended.

Squats

Squats target the muscles of the thighs, hips and buttocks, quads and hamstrings. They are considered a vital exercise for increasing the strength of the legs and glutes, as well as developing core strength as they involve muscles of the lower & upper back, the abdominals, and the shoulders and arms when done in proper form.

To do:

Stand with feet a bit wider than shoulder width apart, keeping the back straight, bend at the knees until thighs become parallel with the floor. (imagine sitting down into a chair without raising the heels) Push with the feet back into a standing position. Hands may be placed behind the head or straight out in front.

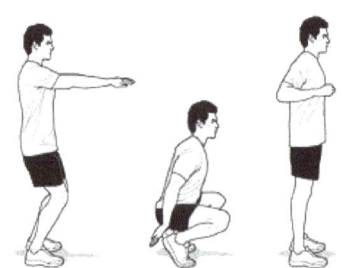

To do:

Walking lunges: Lunge forward with your left thigh parallel to the floor, bring the right leg up to meet, then lunge forward with right thigh parallel to the floor.

Switch Jump Lunges: Lunge forward with your left thigh parallel to the floor, jump up and switch leg positions, landing in a lunge with your right foot forward.

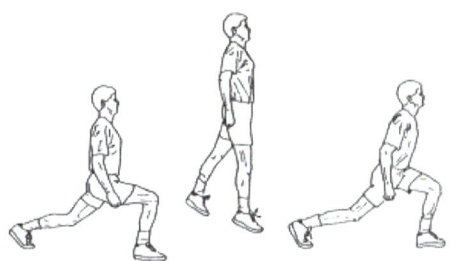

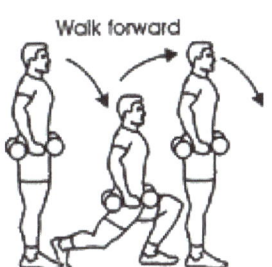

Stair Climbing
Stairs are great for cardio and leg strength. For more advanced trainers you should be running the stairs or setting a stair climber at a higher intensity.

Pull Ups

Pull ups work arms, abdominals, shoulders and chest muscle groups. Many obstacle runs have rope climbs, rings and monkey bars; pull ups will prepare you for these. If you belong to a gym many of them have *assisted pull up* machines. These are a great way for beginners to add this exercise to their workout as they balance out your body weight so that you do not have to pull your entire weight, over time you work up to unassisted pull ups. For home workouts a trx strap comes in handy for assisted pull ups.

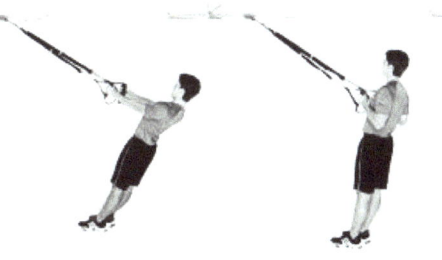

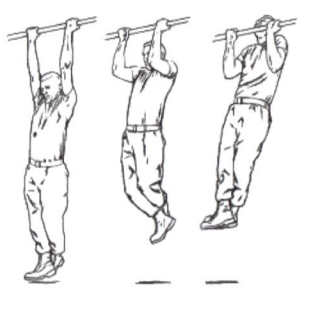

To Do:

Grip the bar with hands shoulder width apart in one of three ways; overhand, underhand, alternative-hand grip. Pull the body up until the chin clears the bar, and finish by lowering the body until your arms and shoulders are fully extended.

Squats

Squats target the muscles of the thighs, hips and buttocks, quads and hamstrings. They are considered a vital exercise for increasing the strength of the legs and glutes, as well as developing core strength as they involve muscles of the lower & upper back, the abdominals, and the shoulders and arms when done in proper form.

To do:

Stand with feet a bit wider than shoulder width apart, keeping the back straight, bend at the knees until thighs become parallel with the floor. (imagine sitting down into a chair without raising the heels) Push with the feet back into a standing position. Hands may be placed behind the head or straight out in front.

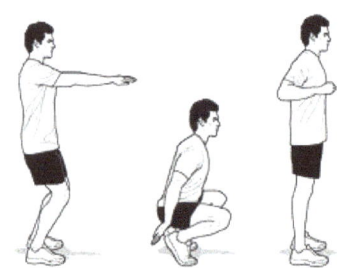

Burpees

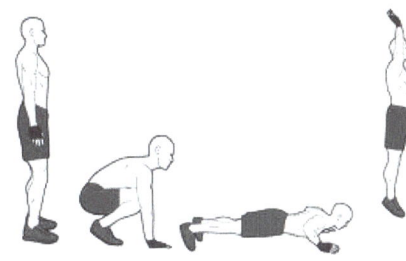

Stand straight with your arms by your side and feet shoulder width apart. Squat down and place your palms face down on the floor in front of you. Kick your legs behind you so you are in a push-up position. Do one push-up, then pull your legs back under you into the squat position, keeping your palms face down on the floor. Stand and then jump in the air, bringing your arms over your head to reach for the ceiling. This completes one burpee.

Military Crawl

This is a great conditioning exercise to prepare you for all those crawl unders through the mud!

To do:
Lie on the ground, using fore arms crawl forward by bringing the knees up beside you one at a time. Keep the head and torso as low to the ground as possible without dragging. Use fore arms and/or hands to pull and toes to push yourself forward.

YOGA

When the schedules say "yoga," complete the following sequence, if you belong to a gym, an hour long yoga or stretch class is a great alternative:

- Mountain Pose
- Forward Fold
- Downward Facing Dog
- Crescent Low Lunge with Eagle Arms on both sides
- Single Pigeon on both sides
- Bound Angle
- Thread the Needle
- Seated Forward Fold

Each of these poses should be held for 30 seconds up to 5 minutes each depending on where you are in your journey. This will be touched on more throughout the guide.

How to do the Yoga Poses!

Mountain Pose

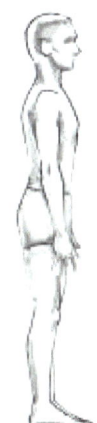

Stand with big toes touching, heels slightly apart. Lift and spread your toes and the balls of your feet, then lay them gently back down. Rock back and forth and side to side; slowly reduce this movement to a standstill, so that your weight is balanced evenly on both feet.

Strength/firm up the legs without locking the knees, then imagine a line of energy all the way up along your inner thighs to your groins, and from there through

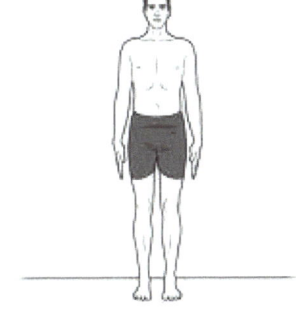

the core of your torso, neck, and out through the crown of your head. Turn the upper thighs slightly inward. Lengthen your tailbone toward the floor and lift the pubis toward the navel.

Press your shoulder blades into your back, then widen them across and release them down your back. Without pushing the ribs forward, lift the top of your sternum straight toward the ceiling. Widen your collarbones. Hang your arms beside the torso with palms facing front.

Balance the crown of your head directly over the center of your pelvis, with the underside of your chin parallel to the floor, throat soft, and the tongue wide and flat on the floor of your mouth. Soften your eyes.

Forward Fold

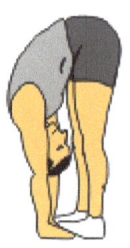

From Standing Mountain inhale and lift the arms overhead without raising the shoulders, on the exhale fold forward from the hips, hands to the ground, moving the torso as one unit.

If you have long hamstrings, you can bring your forehead to your shins. If the hamstrings are short, focus on keeping the torso long. Hunching into a forward bend isn't safe for your lower back and does nothing to lengthen your hamstrings.

With each inhale allow the body to loosen and come out of the fold a little. On each exhale push a little deeper into the fold bringing the chest closer and closer to the shins. Remember to maintain length of the spine without rounding. Hold this pose for 1 to 2 minutes.

On an inhale sweep the arms up with the body returning to standing Mountain Pose.

toward the navel.

Press your shoulder blades into your back, then widen them across and release them down your back. Without pushing the ribs forward, lift the top of your sternum straight toward the ceiling. Widen your collarbones. Hang your arms beside the torso with palms facing front.

Balance the crown of your head directly over the center of your pelvis, with the underside of your chin parallel to the floor, throat soft, and the tongue wide and flat on the floor of your mouth. Soften your eyes.

Forward Fold

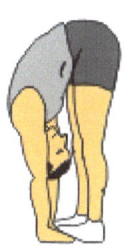

From Standing Mountain inhale and lift the arms overhead without raising the shoulders, on the exhale fold forward from the hips, hands to the ground, moving the torso as one unit.

If you have long hamstrings, you can bring your forehead to your shins. If the hamstrings are short, focus on keeping the torso long. Hunching into a forward bend isn't safe for your lower back and does nothing to lengthen your hamstrings.

With each inhale allow the body to loosen and come out of the fold a little. On each exhale push a little deeper into the fold bringing the chest closer and closer to the shins. Remember to maintain length of the spine without rounding. Hold this pose for 1 to 2 minutes.

On an inhale sweep the arms up with the body returning to standing Mountain Pose.

YOGA

When the schedules say "yoga," complete the following sequence, if you belong to a gym, an hour long yoga or stretch class is a great alternative:

- Mountain Pose
- Forward Fold
- Downward Facing Dog
- Crescent Low Lunge with Eagle Arms on both sides
- Single Pigeon on both sides
- Bound Angle
- Thread the Needle
- Seated Forward Fold

Each of these poses should be held for 30 seconds up to 5 minutes each depending on where you are in your journey. This will be touched on more throughout the guide.

How to do the Yoga Poses!

Mountain Pose

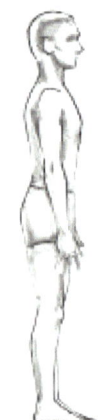

Stand with big toes touching, heels slightly apart. Lift and spread your toes and the balls of your feet, then lay them gently back down. Rock back and forth and side to side; slowly reduce this movement to a standstill, so that your weight is balanced evenly on both feet.

Strength/firm up the legs without locking the knees, then imagine a line of energy all the way up along your inner thighs to your groins, and from there through

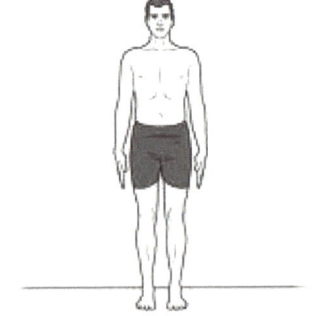

the core of your torso, neck, and out through the crown of your head. Turn the upper thighs slightly inward. Lengthen your tailbone toward the floor and lift the pubis

Downward Facing Dog

Come onto your hands and knees setting the knees directly below the hips and hands slightly forward of your shoulders. Spread your palms, index fingers parallel or slightly turned out, and turn your toes under.

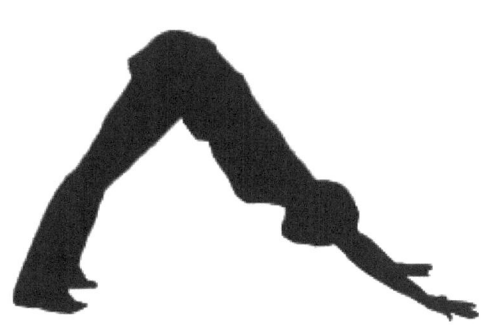

Exhale and lift your knees away from the floor. Lengthen the tailbone towards the ceiling. Inhale as you settle in, with an exhalation, push the thighs back and stretch the heels towards the floor. Straighten your knees being sure not to lock them.

Press the hands firmly into the floor actively using the entire hand. Firm the shoulder blades against your back then widen them and draw toward the tailbone. Keep the head between the upper arms; don't let it hang.

Hold this pose anywhere from 1 to 3 minutes keeping the breath slow and controlled. To come out of the pose bend your right knee, shift into plank and lower right foot between hands. Come up into a lunge.

Crescent Low Lunge with Eagle Arms on both sides

Find your balance and make any adjustments you need to come into a high lunge, keeping the right knee stacked directly over the right ankle. Firm the left thigh and push it up toward the ceiling, holding the left knee straight. Stretch your left heel toward the floor. On an inhale raise the arms over head keeping the shoulders in line with the hips, then release the left knee to the ground.

On an exhale drop the arms out to the side inhale and bring the right arm under left resting the left elbow in the crook of the right arm. Forearms cross to bring palms together. Lift elbows up and away from the body, feeling a slight pull across the shoulder blades. Do not allow the shoulders to creep up towards the ears.

If full eagle arms are not available for you, you may hold each elbow or cross arms in front with hands resting on shoulders.

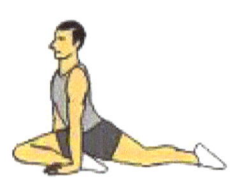

Hold this pose for 5 to 10 deep full breaths. To come out of the pose unwrap arms on an inhale, draw out to sides, then on the exhale bring the body forward allowing the hands to come to rests on either side of your front foot. Push into hands and bring the right foot back to meet the left, on an exhale push back into downward facing dog.

Hold down dog for 3 full breaths to even out the breathing again and repeat with left leg and left arm.

Single Pigeon on both sides

From down dog on an inhale lift the right leg high into the air, exhale as you bring it forward, dropping the left knee to the ground. Slide your right knee forward to the back of your right wrist; at the same time angle your right shin under your torso and bring your right foot to the front of your left knee. The outside of your right shin will now rest on the floor. Slowly slide your left leg back, straightening the knee and descending the front of the thigh to the floor. Lower the outside of your right buttock to the floor. Position the right heel just in front of the left hip.

The right knee can angle slightly to the right, outside the line of the hip. Look back at your left leg. It should extend straight out of the hip (and not be angled off to the left), and rotated slightly inwardly, so its midline presses against the floor. Exhale and lay your torso down on the inner right thigh for a few breaths. You may rest your hand on your hands, or hold yourself up on the forearms. Remember not to strain. It is good to feel a slight pull in the muscles but if it is painful you have gone too far, just release out of the pose a little keeping proper alignment.

Slide your hands back toward the front shin and push your fingertips firmly to the floor. Lift your torso away from the thigh. Lengthen the lower back by pressing your tailbone down and forward.

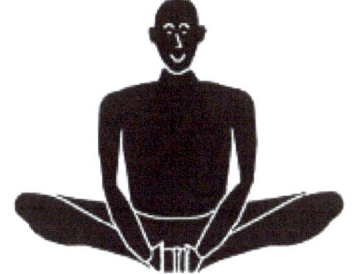

With hands on the floor, curl the toes of your left foot under and push up into plank, bring the right leg back then exhale and lift up and back into Down Dog. Take a few breaths and repeat with the legs reversed for the same length of time.

If your muscles are very tight blocks may be used wherever the body does not touch the floor to encourage proper alignment of the joints. Alignment should always be the focus, do not worry about how far into the stretch you can go. The flexibility will come with practice, patience and time.

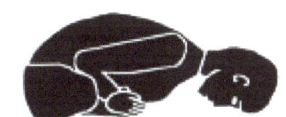

Bound Angle

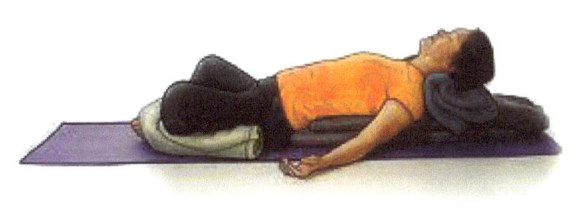

Sit with your legs straight out in front of you, raising your pelvis on a blanket if your hips or groins are tight. Exhale and bend the knees, pulling your heels toward your pelvis, then drop your knees out to the sides and press the soles of your feet together.

Bring your heels as close to your pelvis as you comfortably can, grasp the big toe of each foot. Always keep the outer edges of the feet firmly on the floor. If it isn't possible to hold the toes, clasp each hand around the same-side ankle or shin.

Firm the sacrum and shoulder blades against the back and lengthen the front torso through the top of the sternum.

Never force your knees down, allow gravity to pull the thigh towards the floor.

For a more intense stretch, fold forward over the legs.

For a lighter stretch or for relaxation lie back on the floor. You may wish to support yourself with rolled blankets or blocks. This is a great variation when the guide calls for relaxation yoga.

Whichever position you are in; stay in this pose anywhere from 1 to 5 minutes (longer for relaxation). Then inhale, lift your knees away from the floor, and extend the legs back out in front.

Thread the Needle

From bound angle lie back with knees bent, hip distance apart. Flex the left foot and bring it across to rest on the right knee. Keep the left foot actively flexed to avoid the ankle caving which could cause injury.

Keeping this alignment, pull the right knee in toward your chest; thread your left arm through the triangle between your legs. Without lifting your shoulders off the floor clasp your hands around the back of your right leg or across the shin. If the shoulders round up off the floor use a strap to hold the leg.

Draw the right leg in toward you (making sure to aim it toward your right shoulder and not the center of your chest), simultaneously pressing your left knee away from you.

The goal is to avoid creating tension in the neck and shoulders, the upper body should remain relaxed as the pose works on opening the hips.

Seated Forward Fold

Sit up with legs straight out in front. Shift forward onto the sitting bones by placing your hands just behind the hips, push up so that the buttocks are raised from the ground. Now tilt the pelvis back and settle down.

Tighten your leg muscles pushing the backs of the thighs, calves and heels into the floor; toes toward the ceiling. On an inhale raise the arms above the head lengthening the spine, keeping the shoulders down and back, keeping this length fold forward from the hips as far as you can go releasing the hands to the legs. If it is within your reach, using the index finger and thumb, grasp the big toe. Do not let the heels come off the floor.

Remember the fold comes from the hips, keeping the spine as straight as possible. With each inhale lengthening out the spine from the crown of the head down to the tailbone. With each exhale allow the fold to deepen keeping any length you gain on the inhale.

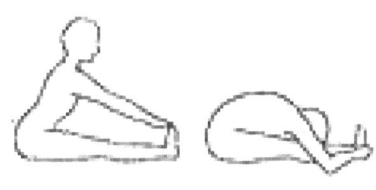

It is ok to allow the body to move slightly to the rhythm of your breath, coming up and extending on an inhale and down on an exhale.

Week 1

This week the focus will be on proper nutrition and will include an introduction into the workout, with beginner running information

Nutritional Basics

Whole foods are any food that occurs naturally, meaning it is not processed in any way. These provide the maximum level of nutrients. All production processes breakdown natural vitamins and minerals; some packaged foods try to add those nutrients back into the product but at a lower quality than was naturally occurring. In most cases the added nutrients are not bioavailable to our bodies (meaning we eliminate them instead of using them). So where ever possible buy and eat foods that come from the earth not from a package!

This week aim to increase the number of fresh vegetables and fruits consumed into your diet. The magic number is 10! 6 servings of vegetables and 4 servings of fruit **every** day.

Remove pop and artificially sweetened food and drinks from your diet.

At the end of this guide are charts you can use to record your progress.

Workout Plan

Definitions:

Aerobic: A pace you set to run at; which allows you to carry out a conversation.

Tempo: This means a bit faster than the aerobic run, you are not expected to keep up a conversation, but can still manage to say a sentence now and then. One way to test: can you huff through one line of a song in the middle of a run? If you cannot get any sound out, you are over exerting yourself, if it is easy and you could sing an entire verse you are at an aerobic pace and need to speed up. Somewhere in between is *tempo*!

Fartlek: Interval running; you do 9 minutes at an aerobic pace then 1 minute at maximum exertion. Repeat this sequence for the duration of your workout.

Follow the chart below for a workout schedule. Days 6 & 7 are rest days to be used anytime throughout the week. On days that you do weight training, unless otherwise stated do the weights first then run. On the yoga days, run first then do yoga.

Never stretch on cold muscles. Do a simple warm up of a few jumping jacks, running on the spot etc. to warm up before a stretch.

If this is your first time **ever** running alternate an aerobic run with walking, building up the running time to eventually cutting it out completely. Example: run 1 minute walk 4, repeat. Run 2 minutes, walk 3 repeat... The goal is to be able to run, at tempo, 5Km in 30 minutes or less within 6 weeks.

This is the week to get to know your body. When running remember to keep testing yourself for aerobic vs. tempo exertion, so that you can pace yourself. If at any time you become dizzy or disoriented stop, what you're doing and breathe! If you feel up to it, continue at a slower pace. Every day is different; your endurance greatly depends on the food you eat, the quality of sleep, and the amount of stress in your day. Some days are much easier to get through than others; the important thing is that you did it. Maybe a bit slower than you wanted but you got through making the next day that much easier.

For this first week "weight training" will consist of the basic exercises provided at the beginning of this guide. "Lunges" are per side i.e. when it reads "10 lunges" this means 10 with the right leg and 10 with the left leg, so that you complete 20 altogether.

If this is your first attempt at running; alternate walking and running throughout the week. With the "walking" times decreasing in length and the "running" times increasing.

If you can already run 5Km introduce fartlek's into your jogs to start pushing yourself a bit harder and further in the allotted timeframe.

If you are a beginner (no running experience) on run days follow:

Run for 1 min. then walk for 3 min. Repeat 8 times.

Day	Cardio	Strength
1	30 minute Aerobic run	5 Burpees, 10 Squats, 5 Burpees 10 Lunges, Pull-ups to failure, 10 Lunges
2	10 minute Jump rope	*Yoga approximately 30 minutes* Mountain Pose Forward Fold Downward Facing Dog Crescent Low Lunge with Eagle Arms on both sides Single Pigeon on both sides Bound Angle Thread the Needle Seated Forward Fold
3	30 minute Aerobic run	5 Burpees, 10 Squats, 5 Burpees 10 Lunges, Pull-ups to failure, 10 Lunges
4	10 minute Jump rope	*Yoga approximately 30 minutes* Mountain Pose Forward Fold Downward Facing Dog Crescent Low Lunge with Eagle Arms on both sides Single Pigeon on both sides Bound Angle Thread the Needle Seated Forward Fold
5	20 minute Aerobic run	5 Burpees, 10 Squats, 5 Burpees 10 Lunges, Pull-ups to failure, 10 Lunges

Use the chart to below to track your nutrition servings throughout the week. The numbers are based on Men and Women ages 30 to 50. If you fall outside of this age range; check your government's food guide to determine the correct numbers for you.

Men	Sunday	Monday	Tuesday	Wednesday	Thursday	Friday	Saturday
Fruits 3-4							
Vegetable 4-6							
Grains 6-8							
Meat/Protein 2-3							
Dairy 1-2							
Water 8-10							

Women	Sunday	Monday	Tuesday	Wednesday	Thursday	Friday	Saturday
Fruits 3-4							
Vegetable 4-6							
Grains 6-8							
Meat/Protein 2-3							
Dairy 1-2							
Water 6-8							

Use this space each week to record any thoughts and/or feelings about your training.

_____

_____

_____

_____

_____

_____

_____

_____

_____

_____

_____

Week 2

This week increase your lean proteins, replace things like luncheon meets with chicken breast, try steaming or baking fresh fish. Bake a whole chicken, skin removed, cut the meat away from the bones and refrigerate for quick meals over the next couple days. Use the chicken for a quick protein fix over a salad, toss with vegetables into a quick pasta, fold into an egg-white omelet...the possibilities are endless!

Beginner Run Variation:

Run for 1 min. then walk for 2 min. Repeat 8 times.

Day	Cardio	Strength
1	10 minute aerobic run 5 minutes tempo run 5 minutes aerobic run or walk	10 Burpees, 15 Squats, 10 Burpees 15 Lunges, Pull-ups to failure, 15 Lunges Military crawl 3 minutes
2	10 minute Jump Rope	Yoga approximately 30 minutes Mountain Pose Forward Fold Downward Facing Dog Crescent Low Lunge with Eagle Arms on both sides Single Pigeon on both sides Bound Angle Thread the Needle Seated Forward Fold
3	30 minute Aerobic run	10 Burpees, 15 Squats, 10 Burpees 15 Lunges, Pull-ups to failure, 15 Lunges Military crawl 3 minutes
4	45 minute Treadmill: alternate hills and flat terrain Walking and running If you are running outside choose a route with hills, if no hills are available, every 10 minutes do walking lunges for 2 to 5 minutes	Yoga approximately 30 minutes Mountain Pose Forward Fold Downward Facing Dog Crescent Low Lunge with Eagle Arms on both sides Single Pigeon on both sides Bound Angle Thread the Needle Seated Forward Fold
5	10 minute Jump Rope	10 Burpees, 15 Squats, 10 Burpees 15 Lunges, Pull-ups to failure, 15 Lunges Military crawl 3 minutes

Use the chart to below to track your nutrition servings throughout the week. The numbers are based on Men and Women ages 30 to 50. If you fall outside of this age range; check your government's food guide to determine the correct numbers for you.

Men	Sunday	Monday	Tuesday	Wednesday	Thursday	Friday	Saturday
Fruits 3-4							
Vegetable 4-6							
Grains 6-8							
Meat/Protein 2-3							
Dairy 1-2							
Water 8-10							

Women	Sunday	Monday	Tuesday	Wednesday	Thursday	Friday	Saturday
Fruits 3-4							
Vegetable 4-6							
Grains 6-8							
Meat/Protein 2-3							
Dairy 1-2							
Water 6-8							

Use the chart to below to track your nutrition servings throughout the week. The numbers are based on Men and Women ages 30 to 50. If you fall outside of this age range; check your government's food guide to determine the correct numbers for you.

Men	Sunday	Monday	Tuesday	Wednesday	Thursday	Friday	Saturday
Fruits 3-4							
Vegetable 4-6							
Grains 6-8							
Meat/Protein 2-3							
Dairy 1-2							
Water 8-10							

Women	Sunday	Monday	Tuesday	Wednesday	Thursday	Friday	Saturday
Fruits 3-4							
Vegetable 4-6							
Grains 6-8							
Meat/Protein 2-3							
Dairy 1-2							
Water 6-8							

Use this space each week to record any thoughts and/or feelings about your training.

Week 4

Take this week to examine your mental attitude. Answer the following questions, being fully honest with yourself. Each day this week ask yourself these questions:

- How are you feeling? Physically? Emotionally?
- What have you found the hardest so far? The easiest?
- Are you having trouble getting through the workouts? Or finding the motivation to workout?
- Have you been able to cut sugary drinks and foods from your diet?

If you are finding something particularly hard take a few minutes to examine why. Try changing the mental mantra. Example: "I just can't push myself past 5 minutes of running" change it to "Today I WILL run for 6 minutes, I know I CAN do it, look how far I have come". Remember to say it with conviction!

This week will be a bit of a break. The last 3 weeks you really pushed it, making progress each day. The body needs time to absorb and repair all that is new.

Beginner Run Variation:

Run for 2 min. then walk for 1 min. Repeat 8 times.

Day	Cardio	Strength
1	10 minute aerobic run 5 minute jump rope 10 minute aerobic run	10 Burpees, 15 weighted Squats, 10 Burpees 15 weighted lunges, Pull-ups to failure, 15 weighted lunges Military crawl 4 minutes
2	Recovery day, no aerobic exercise. Use the yoga portion to relax and release tension from hard worked muscles.	Mountain Pose Forward Fold Downward Facing Dog Crescent Low Lunge with Eagle Arms on both sides Single Pigeon on both sides Bound Angle Thread the Needle Seated Forward Fold
3	15 minute Jump rope	10 Burpees, 10 weighted Squats, 10 Burpees 10 weighted lunges, Pull-ups to failure, 10 weighted lunges
4	Recovery day, no aerobic exercise. Use the yoga portion to relax and release tension from hard worked muscles.	Mountain Pose Forward Fold Downward Facing Dog Crescent Low Lunge with Eagle Arms on both sides Single Pigeon on both sides Bound Angle Thread the Needle Seated Forward Fold
5	30 minute Treadmill: alternate hills and flat terrain Aerobic run	10 Burpees, 15 weighted Squats, 10 Burpees 15 weighted lunges, Pull-ups to failure, 15 weighted lunges

Use the chart to below to track your nutrition servings throughout the week. The numbers are based on Men and Women ages 30 to 50. If you fall outside of this age range; check your government's food guide to determine the correct numbers for you.

Men	Sunday	Monday	Tuesday	Wednesday	Thursday	Friday	Saturday
Fruits 3-4							
Vegetable 4-6							
Grains 6-8							
Meat/Protein 2-3							
Dairy 1-2							
Water 8-10							

Women	Sunday	Monday	Tuesday	Wednesday	Thursday	Friday	Saturday
Fruits 3-4							
Vegetable 4-6							
Grains 6-8							
Meat/Protein 2-3							
Dairy 1-2							
Water 6-8							

Use this space each week to record any thoughts and/or feelings about your training.

_____

_____

_____

_____

_____

_____

_____

_____

_____

_____

Week 5

How are you feeling after the recovery week? Are you ready to get back to business?

This week really try to push the runs. If you have been walking for short duration push yourself a bit harder to get the full run in. If you need the walking time shorten the run length so on the 30 minute run days; run for 20 instead of walking in between. On the 45 minute run days, try to push out 30 minutes of running time without walking in between.

Beginner Run Variation:

Run for 3 min. then walk for 1 min. Repeat 8 times.

Day	Cardio	Strength
1	10 minute aerobic run 15 minute tempo run 5 minute aerobic run	10 Burpees, 15 weighted squats, 10 Burpees 15 weighted lunges, Pull-ups to failure, 15 weighted lunges Military crawl 4 minutes
2	45 minute Aerobic run Broken up with jump rope in 2 minute intervals Ie. Run 13 skip 2	Mountain Pose Forward Fold Downward Facing Dog Crescent Low Lunge with Eagle Arms on both sides Single Pigeon on both sides Bound Angle Thread the Needle Seated Forward Fold
3	30 minutes Aerobic run	10 Burpees, 15 weighted Squats, 10 Burpees 15 weighted lunges, Pull-ups to failure, 15 weighted lunges Military crawl 4 minutes
4	45 minute Treadmill: alternate hills and flat terrain Aerobic run If you are running outside choose a route with hills, if no hills are available, every 10 minutes do walking lunges for 2 to 5 minutes	Mountain Pose Forward Fold Downward Facing Dog Crescent Low Lunge with Eagle Arms on both sides Single Pigeon on both sides Bound Angle Thread the Needle Seated Forward Fold
5	20 minutes Jog with fartlek's 10 minute jump rope	10 Burpees, 15 weighted Squats, 10 Burpees 15 weighted lunges, Pull-ups to failure, 15 weighted lunges Military crawl 4 minutes

Use the chart to below to track your nutrition servings throughout the week. The numbers are based on Men and Women ages 30 to 50. If you fall outside of this age range; check your government's food guide to determine the correct numbers for you.

Men	Sunday	Monday	Tuesday	Wednesday	Thursday	Friday	Saturday
Fruits 3-4							
Vegetable 4-6							
Grains 6-8							
Meat/Protein 2-3							
Dairy 1-2							
Water 8-10							

Women	Sunday	Monday	Tuesday	Wednesday	Thursday	Friday	Saturday
Fruits 3-4							
Vegetable 4-6							
Grains 6-8							
Meat/Protein 2-3							
Dairy 1-2							
Water 6-8							

Week 6

By now you should be running 5km without stopping. For most obstacle runs this is sufficient stamina to complete a course. That said, this is not enough stamina if you are trying to finish in record time! However the fun of obstacle runs is of course the obstacles! Which, while difficult, also provide a rest period and allow for some water & washroom breaks in the longer runs (such as Tough Mudder)

Over the past 6 weeks we have been slowly increasing weights and resistance while really pushing the stamina/running portion of the training. Now we will shift the focus to push harder at weight training while maintaining and/or slowly building the running portion.

Weight Training

Additional Exercises

Biceps Curl: Position 2 dumbbells on either side, palms facing in; with elbows to sides, raise one dumbbell and rotate forearm until forearm is vertical and palm faces shoulder. Lower to original position and repeat with opposite arm. Continue to alternate between sides.

Single Arm Pullover: Lying with your back on a bench and with your feet on the floor, hold a dumbbell in one hand and point the elbow of this same arm toward the ceiling. With your other hand, grasp the inside of your elbow on the weighted arm to stabilize the motion. Extend your arm until it is pointing straight up, then lower it back down near your face. To build muscle use weights that allow you to complete 6 to 8 reps, to tone use weight that allows you to complete 12 to 15 reps.

Push Ups: Lie on the ground with hands placed shoulder width apart. Keeping the body straight, bend at the elbows and lower body to the ground. Raise body up off the ground by extending the arms. Keep the core strong, do not let the stomach fall.

Shoulder Press & Squat: As in weighted squats hold the "toning" weights in front of your body shoulder distance apart. Keeping the back straight allow the weights to hang in front on the squat, as you rise lifts the weights to shoulder height, once standing lift the weights overhead then return to starting position and repeat.

Dips: Sit on the edge of a solid chair or bench and hold the front edge of the seat on both sides of your body. Your knuckles should be facing forward, not turned to the sides, feet firmly planted to the floor. Push yourself off the seat and lower your buttocks below it until your arms form a 90-degree angle, then push back into starting position (making sure not to lock the elbows). Repeat until you can't do any more.

Plank: place hands on ground shoulder width apart extend legs straight out behind you so that toes are pressed firmly into the ground and weight is distributed evenly between hands and feet. Keep core muscles contracted, body in a straight line, do not let the belly drop, this creates a sway in the lower back and can cause injury. Imagine you are being pulled by the crown of your head straight out in front and by the heels of the feet straight out behind in opposing directions. Hold for 30 seconds, then shift weight to the left hand for side plank.

Side Plank: From plank position shift onto the outside edge of your left foot, and stack your right foot on top. As you turn your body to the right, swing your right hand onto your right hip; supporting the weight of your body on the outer left foot and left hand. Hold for 30 seconds watch where you are going and return right hand to ground under right shoulder turning back into plank

Tips to prepare you for the differing terrains:

- Outside running - head for some country roads.
- Alternate running on the grass, and road.
- Try to plan the route on some dirt roads!
- See a tree with low branches stop and do as many pull-ups as possible.
- Military crawl through the gully
- Run a fartlek then do 20 walking lunges through tall grass

- Head for a park, run the perimeter, then run the equipment as an obstacle, climb, crawl, jump, balance...repeat for 1 hour!

Note About Weights

For the next few weeks it would be handy to have 2 sets of weights one to tone and one to build. The ideal weight for building your muscles is a weight that you can push out 7 to 8 reps. The last rep should be *very* hard! The toning weights should be light enough that you can do 12 to 15 reps, but not so heavy that you feel you have trouble pushing out the last rep.

Under the strength headings you will see "max weight", and "light weight", when strength training muscles needs both a building period and a toning period. The days of "light weight" the weight is lower but the reps are higher to promote toning of the muscles groups.

Beginner Run Variation:

Run for 4 min. then walk for 1 min. Repeat 6 times.

Day	Cardio	Strength
1	15 minute Aerobic run 10 minute Jump rope 15 minute Aerobic run	*Max weights* 10 Burpees 20 weighted shoulder press & squat 20 weighted lunges Pull-ups to failure Biceps curl 3 sets of 8 to build Single arm pullover 3 sets of 8 to build 20 push-ups Dips to failure
2	45 to 60 minutes Divide the time between Stair climbing Aerobic run Lunges (@ the gym: treadmill, stair machine, elliptical)	Mountain Pose Forward Fold Downward Facing Dog Crescent Low Lunge with Eagle Arms on both sides Plank, left side plank, plank, right side plank, plank (hold 20 to 30 seconds each pose) Single Pigeon on both sides Bound Angle Thread the Needle Seated Forward Fold
3	10 minute aerobic run Do ½ of the strength training 10 minute aerobic run Other ½ of strength training 10 minutes Aerobic run	*Light weight* 10 Burpees 20 weighted shoulder press & squat 20 weighted lunges Pull-ups to failure Biceps curl 3 sets of 15 to tone Single arm pullover 3 sets of 15 to tone 20 push-ups Dips to failure
4	45 to 60 minutes Divide the time between Stair climbing Aerobic run Lunges (@ the gym: treadmill, stair machine, elliptical)	Mountain Pose Forward Fold Downward Facing Dog Crescent Low Lunge with Eagle Arms on both sides Plank, left side plank, plank, right side plank, plank (hold 20 to 30 seconds each pose) Single Pigeon on both sides Bound Angle Thread the Needle Seated Forward Fold
5	30 minutes Jog with fartlek's	*Max weights* 10 Burpees 20 weighted shoulder press & squat 20 weighted lunges Pull-ups to failure Biceps curl 3 sets of 8 to build Single arm pullover 3 sets of 8 to build 20 push-ups Dips to failure

Use the chart to below to track your nutrition servings throughout the week. The numbers are based on Men and Women ages 30 to 50. If you fall outside of this age range; check your government's food guide to determine the correct numbers for you.

Men	Sunday	Monday	Tuesday	Wednesday	Thursday	Friday	Saturday
Fruits 3-4							
Vegetable 4-6							
Grains 6-8							
Meat/Protein 2-3							
Dairy 1-2							
Water 8-10							

Women	Sunday	Monday	Tuesday	Wednesday	Thursday	Friday	Saturday
Fruits 3-4							
Vegetable 4-6							
Grains 6-8							
Meat/Protein 2-3							
Dairy 1-2							
Water 6-8							

Use this space each week to record any thoughts and/or feelings about your training.

_____

_____

_____

_____

_____

_____

_____

_____

_____

_____

_____

_____

Week 7

Beginner Run Variation:

Run for 6 min. then walk for 1 min. Repeat 5 times.

Day	Cardio	Strength
1	15 minute Aerobic run 10 minute Jump rope 15 minute Aerobic run	*Max weights* 10 Burpees 20 weighted shoulder press & squat 20 weighted lunges Pull-ups to failure Biceps curl 3 sets of 8 to build Single arm pullover 3 sets of 8 to build 20 push-ups Dips to failure
2	45 minutes Divide the time between Stair climbing Aerobic run Lunges (@ the gym: 15 minutes each, treadmill, stair machine, elliptical)	Mountain Pose Forward Fold Downward Facing Dog Crescent Low Lunge with Eagle Arms on both sides Plank, left side plank, plank, right side plank, plank (hold 20 to 30 seconds each pose) Single Pigeon on both sides Bound Angle Thread the Needle Seated Forward Fold
3	10 minute aerobic run Do ½ of the strength training 10 minute aerobic run Other ½ of strength training 10 minutes Aerobic run	*Light weight* 10 Burpees 20 weighted shoulder press & squat 20 weighted lunges Pull-ups to failure Biceps curl 3 sets of 15 to tone Single arm pullover 3 sets of 15 to tone 20 push-ups Dips to failure
4	30 minutes Divide the time between Stair climbing Aerobic run Lunges (@ the gym: treadmill, stair machine, elliptical)	Mountain Pose Forward Fold Downward Facing Dog Crescent Low Lunge with Eagle Arms on both sides Plank, left side plank, plank, right side plank, plank (hold 20 to 30 seconds each pose) Single Pigeon on both sides Bound Angle Thread the Needle Seated Forward Fold
5	15 minute Jump rope	*Max weights* 10 Burpees 20 weighted shoulder press & squat 20 weighted lunges Pull-ups to failure Biceps curl 3 sets of 8 to build Single arm pullover 3 sets of 8 to build 20 push-ups Dips to failure

Use the chart to below to track your nutrition servings throughout the week. The numbers are based on Men and Women ages 30 to 50. If you fall outside of this age range; check your government's food guide to determine the correct numbers for you.

Men	Sunday	Monday	Tuesday	Wednesday	Thursday	Friday	Saturday
Fruits 3-4							
Vegetable 4-6							
Grains 6-8							
Meat/Protein 2-3							
Dairy 1-2							
Water 8-10							

Women	Sunday	Monday	Tuesday	Wednesday	Thursday	Friday	Saturday
Fruits 3-4							
Vegetable 4-6							
Grains 6-8							
Meat/Protein 2-3							
Dairy 1-2							
Water 6-8							

Use this space each week to record any thoughts and/or feelings about your training.

_____

_____

_____

_____

_____

_____

_____

_____

_____

_____

_____

Week 8

Can you increase your *Max Weight* this week? Try the weighted reps a couple pounds heavier, keeping the *Light Weights* the same.

Beginner Run Variation:

Run for 8 min. then walk for 1 min. Repeat 4 times

Day	Cardio	Strength
1	15 minute Aerobic run 10 minute Jump rope 15 minute Aerobic run	*Max Weight* 15 Burpees 20 weighted shoulder press & squat 20 weighted lunges Pull-ups to failure Biceps curl 3 sets of 8 to build Single arm pullover 3 sets of 8 to build 20 push-ups Dips to failure
2	45 to 60 minutes Divide the time between Stair climbing Aerobic run Lunges (@ the gym: treadmill, stair machine, elliptical)	Mountain Pose Forward Fold Downward Facing Dog Crescent Low Lunge with Eagle Arms on both sides Plank, left side plank, plank, right side plank, plank (hold 20 to 30 seconds each pose) Single Pigeon on both sides Bound Angle Thread the Needle Seated Forward Fold
3	15 minute aerobic run Do ½ of the strength training 10 minute aerobic run Other ½ of strength training 15 minutes Aerobic run	*Light weight* 10 Burpees 20 weighted shoulder press & squat 20 weighted lunges Pull-ups to failure Biceps curl 3 sets of 15 to tone Single arm pullover 3 sets of 15 to tone 20 push-ups Dips to failure
4	30 minutes Divide the time between Stair climbing Aerobic run Lunges (@ the gym: treadmill, stair machine, elliptical set at high intensity)	Mountain Pose Forward Fold Downward Facing Dog Crescent Low Lunge with Eagle Arms on both sides Plank, left side plank, plank, right side plank, plank (hold 20 to 30 seconds each pose) Single Pigeon on both sides Bound Angle Thread the Needle Seated Forward Fold
5	15 minute Jump rope	*Max weight* 15 Burpees 20 weighted shoulder press & squat 20 weighted lunges Pull-ups to failure Biceps curl 3 sets of 8 to build Single arm pullover 3 sets of 8 to build 20 push-ups Dips to failure

Use the chart to below to track your nutrition servings throughout the week. The numbers are based on Men and Women ages 30 to 50. If you fall outside of this age range; check your government's food guide to determine the correct numbers for you.

Men	Sunday	Monday	Tuesday	Wednesday	Thursday	Friday	Saturday
Fruits 3-4							
Vegetable 4-6							
Grains 6-8							
Meat/Protein 2-3							
Dairy 1-2							
Water 8-10							

Women	Sunday	Monday	Tuesday	Wednesday	Thursday	Friday	Saturday
Fruits 3-4							
Vegetable 4-6							
Grains 6-8							
Meat/Protein 2-3							
Dairy 1-2							
Water 6-8							

Use this space each week to record any thoughts and/or feelings about your training.

_____

_____

_____

_____

_____

_____

_____

_____

_____

_____

_____

Week 9

This is the last week of full training so make it a good one! If you have not had a chance to run outside yet make sure to do so this week. Your body needs to know what it will be up against on race day! Rain or shine; get out there!

Day	Cardio	Strength
1	20 minute aerobic run 10 minute tempo run 5 minute aerobic run	*Max Weight* 15 Burpees 20 weighted shoulder press & squat 20 weighted lunges Pull-ups to failure Biceps curl 3 sets of 8 to build Single arm pullover 3 sets of 8 to build 20 push-ups Dips to failure
2	45 minute Aerobic run	Mountain Pose Forward Fold Downward Facing Dog Crescent Low Lunge with Eagle Arms on both sides Plank, left side plank, plank, right side plank, plank (hold 20 to 30 seconds each pose) Single Pigeon on both sides Bound Angle Thread the Needle Seated Forward Fold
3	10 minute aerobic run Do ½ of the strength training 10 minute aerobic run Other ½ of strength training 10 minutes Aerobic run	*Light weight* 10 Burpees 20 weighted shoulder press & squat 20 weighted lunges Pull-ups to failure Biceps curl 3 sets of 15 to tone Single arm pullover 3 sets of 15 to tone 20 push-ups Dips to failure
4	45 minute Treadmill: alternate hills and flat terrain Aerobic run If you are running outside choose a route with hills, if no hills are available, every 10 minutes do walking lunges for 2 to 5 minutes	Mountain Pose Forward Fold Downward Facing Dog Crescent Low Lunge with Eagle Arms on both sides Plank, left side plank, plank, right side plank, plank (hold 20 to 30 seconds each pose) Single Pigeon on both sides Bound Angle Thread the Needle Seated Forward Fold
5	15 minute Jump rope	*Max weight* 15 Burpees 20 weighted shoulder press & squat 20 weighted lunges Pull-ups to failure Biceps curl 3 sets of 8 to build Single arm pullover 3 sets of 8 to build 20 push-ups Dips to failure

Use the chart to below to track your nutrition servings throughout the week. The numbers are based on Men and Women ages 30 to 50. If you fall outside of this age range; check your government's food guide to determine the correct numbers for you.

Men	Sunday	Monday	Tuesday	Wednesday	Thursday	Friday	Saturday
Fruits 3-4							
Vegetable 4-6							
Grains 6-8							
Meat/Protein 2-3							
Dairy 1-2							
Water 8-10							

Women	Sunday	Monday	Tuesday	Wednesday	Thursday	Friday	Saturday
Fruits 3-4							
Vegetable 4-6							
Grains 6-8							
Meat/Protein 2-3							
Dairy 1-2							
Water 6-8							

Week 10

Week of the Event

Congratulations, you made it! This week is about pampering yourself to ensure proper nutrition, flexibility, hydration and rest before your chosen event.

Monday

Light jog – 20 to 30 minutes at any pace you like. Don't push yourself today, keep it easy but make sure you get the exercise in. Finish the run with a half hour light yoga set.

Tuesday

Take 1 hour and do the light weight set from the previous week.

Wednesday

Relaxation yoga, do the yoga set holding each pose for 2 to 5 minutes. Pamper your muscles let them sink slowly into each pose, use block or bolsters to support the joints where needed. This session is about relaxation not over stretching.

Thursday

Relax! Do some light yoga if you desire or even a light run, no more than 3 Km!

Friday

Use the day to stay hydrated, drink at least 2 litres of water today. The best way to ensure proper hydration is to add fresh lemon or lime to a 2 litre jug of filtered water. The citrus allows the water to be more readily available for uptake into your cells. Finish drinking by dinner time to allow time for absorption. You don't want a sloshy stomach on event day!

Try to avoid pre-event parties alcohol dehydrates the body, save it for after the event!

The nutritional focus of the day is carbohydrates. Complex carbs are the best energy source for aerobic exertion. Also orange vegetables as they contain higher amounts of B group vitamins which are responsible for stress reduction and energy production. The *Caribbean Curry Stew* (recipe found at the end of this guide) would be a great option for dinner.

Saturday

Event day!

Don't forget your bananas, potassium in bananas help to prevent muscle cramps during and after the run. Most races provide them or a power bar after the event; however they have been known to run short especially if you are racing towards the end of the day, so it is always helpful to bring your own.

On colder days bring extra pants, leg warmers, heavy socks for after race. In colder weather muscles cool down too fast leading to cramps and muscle pain. By encouraging the muscles to cool down at a slower rate you can prevent post-race pain.

Warm up before your start time with small bursts of energy such as jumping jacks, push-ups, running on the spot, lunges and squats, but don't exert yourself! Do not stretch beforehand unless your muscles are nice and warm. It is ok to leave the stretching for after the run.

Cool down from the event by doing some stretches; this will help to keep the muscles loose instead of tightening up.

Good luck and remember to have a blast!

Use the chart to below to track your nutrition servings throughout the week. The numbers are based on Men and Women ages 30 to 50. If you fall outside of this age range; check your government's food guide to determine the correct numbers for you.

Men	Sunday	Monday	Tuesday	Wednesday	Thursday	Friday	Saturday
Fruits 3-4							
Vegetable 4-6							
Grains 6-8							
Meat/Protein 2-3							
Dairy 1-2							
Water 8-10							

Women	Sunday	Monday	Tuesday	Wednesday	Thursday	Friday	Saturday
Fruits 3-4							
Vegetable 4-6							
Grains 6-8							
Meat/Protein 2-3							
Dairy 1-2							
Water 6-8							

Use this space each week to record any thoughts and/or feelings about your training.

_____

_____

_____

_____

_____

_____

_____

_____

_____

_____

_____

Recipes

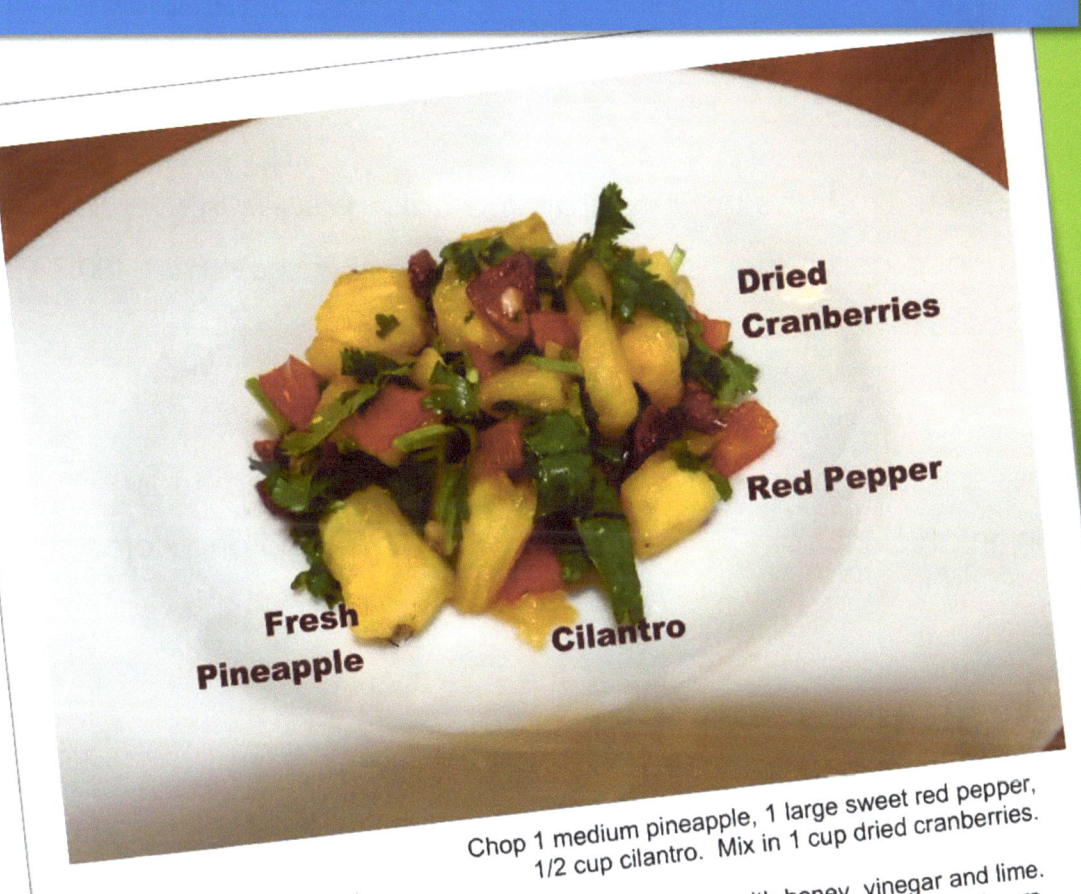

Dried Cranberries

Red Pepper

Cilantro

Fresh Pineapple

Chop 1 medium pineapple, 1 large sweet red pepper, 1/2 cup cilantro. Mix in 1 cup dried cranberries.

Toss with honey, vinegar and lime. Let sit 1 hour up to 48 hours.

1 tbs. honey
3 tbs. apple cider vinegar
squeeze of fresh lime

Amounts can be adjusted to taste preferences.

This "salsa" is a great accompaniment to steamed fish, grilled chicken breast or with some fresh flat breads!

www.NaturalJenn.com

Steamed Fish with Fresh Mango Salsa

Fresh cod fillets
Olive oil (to brush pan)

1 cup chopped Cilantro
2 large mangos, ripe but firm, diced

1 quart cherry tomatoes, halved
1 red pepper, cut into small pieces
1 red onion, chopped
2 tablespoons apple cider vinegar

If you have a steamer, olive oil brush the bottom and place cod into pan, steam for 20 minutes or until cooked.

No steamer? No problem! Brush the bottom of a large baking pan with a small amount of olive oil. Place cod in pan and bake in a pre-heated oven at 400 degrees Fahrenheit for 20 minutes or until cooked.

Meanwhile prepare salsa: in a large bowl mix cilantro, chopped mango, tomato, pepper, onion and vinegar. This may be made beforehand and stored in the refrigerator.

To serve: plate cod and top with a generous helping of salsa!

Caribbean Curry Stew

2 firm mangos, chopped
1 or 2 medium sized sweet potatoes
2 red peppers
2 or 3 medium sized potatoes
1 can black eyed peas
1 cup cut up carrots or whole baby carrots
4 to 6 bone-in, skinless chicken breasts
3 tbsp. curry powder

Pepper to taste
6 buds of garlic
1 large onion, diced
1 can coconut milk (optional)
Water to cover

2 cups chopped spinach
1 cup chopped cilantro

Place chicken, onion, garlic, black eyed peas, and all vegetables except spinach & cilantro into a large baking pan or slow cooker Mix curry powder with coconut milk (if not using mix with 1 cup water) pour over chicken/vegetable mixture. Pour in enough water to almost cover. Cook in oven for 1 1/2 hours at 350 degrees or until chicken is cooked through and potatoes are tender. Or cook on "stew" setting of slow cooker.

To serve divide spinach evenly in bottom of bowls, spoon stew over spinach and garnish with chopped cilantro.

Anything Muffins

These muffins make a great breakfast or quick snack, the more you add the healthier they become.

Ingredients:

1 cup oats (or any grain/cereal)   ½ tsp. baking soda
1 cup flour (whole wheat preferable)   ½ tsp. salt
¾ cup organic sugar   1 egg beaten
1 tsp. baking powder   ¼ melted butter
1 cup liquid (sour milk, orange juice, mashed banana, almond milk...)
Optional – ¾ cup of any dry ingredient such as dry fruit, chocolate chips, nuts...

Preheat oven to 400 degrees.

Combine grain with liquid. In a separate bowl mix all other dry ingredients. Add melted butter and egg to liquid/grain mixture, fold wet and dry ingredient together until moist. Divide evenly into 12 muffins tins bake for 15 to 22 minutes.

Fun Variations!

Banana, Bran, Walnut – fold in ¾ cup of chopped walnuts and use mashed bananas as the liquid (3 works best) and bran for grain.

Orange, Date, Bran – fold in ¾ cup chopped dates. Use orange juice for liquid and bran for grain.

Oatmeal, Blueberry – fold in 1 cup fresh blueberries. Use steel cut oats as grain and sour cream for liquid, add in 1 tsp. vanilla with liquid.

Juicer pulp – If you have a juicer the fibrous pulp that remains can be used in these muffins. Sift through the pulp to remove larger chunks. This tends to make the muffins heavier; adding an extra ½ teaspoon of baking soda will combat this.

Have fun trying new combinations. Fruit granola cereals make a great addition as a grain. If using prepackaged cereals decrease sugar to 1/3 cup.

Just remember to keep the ratio of 1:1:1, (liquid : flour : grain)

Faux Fried Chicken

Leaving the bone in chicken adds flavor however if your prefer boneless, skinless chicken breasts work great too! You can even cut the chicken into strips to eat as a healthier version of chicken fingers. This is handy if you have a hard time judging portion size. A smaller girl would only eat half of a chicken breast or 2 strips; whereas a larger man would eat a whole breast or 4 strips.

4 bone-in skinless chicken breasts
½ cup favorite creamy salad dressing (try to find a healthy choice dressing without high fructose corn syrup)
½ bread crumbs

1 cup crushed corn flakes
¼ cup grated parmesan cheese
Pepper to taste
1 tsp. Italian herbs

Coat chicken in salad dressing and refrigerate for 2 hours or overnight.

Combine all dry ingredients, toss coated chicken and place on baking sheet. Bake in oven at 350 F for 1 hour until chicken is cooked through and coating is crispy!

Enjoy with a salad of fresh vegetables for a complete meal.

Butternut Squash Salad

Can be enjoyed as a main dish for vegetarians or as a side with meat of your choice. As with any recipe play with it and have fun adding your favorite raw vegetables for greater nutritional value.

½ butternut squash, cubed (about 2 cups small cubes)
1 tbsp. olive oil
1 cup brown or red rice
½ cup chopped parsley
1 cup shredded Napa cabbage

½ cup of fruit and seed mix (make your own: mix ½ cup each of sunflower seeds, dried cranberries, dried papaya, sliced almonds)
Balsamic vinegar

Toss diced squash with olive oil and bake in 350 F oven for 20 minutes or until tender. Cook rice as directed on package. Let rice & squash cool.

Toss cooked rice, squash, cabbage, parsley, fruit & seed mix.

To serve sprinkle with balsamic vinegar.

Cure-all Drink!

Be warned this tea packs a real kick! Adding a bit of honey to your cup helps it go down; but the health benefits are well worth the burning!

This tea helps flush out the lymphatic system and reduce swelling. It is a great anti-inflammatory and may help with many health issues (headache, sore throat, cough due to colds or bronchitis, stomach upset, supports heart health...). It is also a great cleansing detox for the entire body.

The anti-inflammatory properties of this beverage are great for post run; enjoy the night of the race and the morning after to help ease sore muscles.

4 Lemons
2-3 inch piece of fresh ginger root
1-2 inch piece of fresh turmeric root (optional)
1-2 dashes of cayenne (or juice 1/2 a habanero or jalapeño pepper)

In a juicer, juice your ginger root, turmeric, and lemons.

If you do not have a juicer crush the ginger root and turmeric root and let soak in 2 cups boiling water for 1 hour. Strain out the roots, then squeeze in the lemons.

Refrigerate until ready to serve.

To serve pour about 1/3 cup of juice into a cup (you can add 1 tsp. of honey) fill the cup with any temperature water you prefer (to ease a sore throat add hot water, for a refresher add cold!)

Will last about 5 days in the fridge.

Left Over Roast Chicken Salad

Remove roasted chicken from bones, chop into small chunks. Discard skin and bones.

1 – 2 Tbsp. natural yogurt
Juice from ½ lemon
¼ cup sunflower or pumpkin seeds
½ - 1 cup grapes cut in half (depending on amount of chicken leftover)
¼ cup dried cranberries
1 tbsp fresh chopped mint leaves

Toss all ingredients together, salt & pepper to taste. Lemonaise can be used in place of the yogurt and lemon. Enjoy with your favourite bread or cracker.

Endive leaves are a nice alternative to bread if you are avoiding gluten or just want a lighter meal.

About the Author

Dr. Jennifer Heard is a Doctor of Natural Medicine specializing in Yoga Therapy and Clinical Nutrition to promote healing in a natural way.

This guide was developed while the author and her husband trained for Tough Mudder. They found at the end of the course they were in better shape than the rest of the group and their recovery time was faster over the days following the course.

"I hope you have as much fun training as I did; wherever possible make it personal! The feeling of actually completing an obstacle run is amazing, something I never thought I could accomplish"

Dr. Jennifer Heard
BSc, DNM, PHS, TY, PTS